Turmeric

Spices of Life

Barbara Wexler, MPH

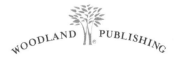

WOODLAND PUBLISHING

For permissions, ordering information, or bulk quantity discounts, contact:
Woodland Publishing, Salt Lake City, Utah
Visit our Web site: *www.woodlandpublishing.com*
Toll-free number: (800) 777-BOOK

The information in this book is for educational purposes only and is not recommended as a means of diagnosing or treating an illness. All matters concerning physical and mental health should be supervised by a health practitioner knowledgeable in treating that particular condition. Neither the publisher nor the author directly or indirectly dispenses medical advice, nor do they prescribe any remedies or assume any responsibility for those who choose to treat themselves.

Cataloging-in-Publication data is available from the Library of Congress.

ISBN: 978-1-58054-183-1

Printed in the United States of America

Contents

> *There is also a vegetable that has all the properties of true saffron, as well as the smell and the color, and yet it is not really saffron.*
> — *Marco Polo, during his tour of China in 1280*

A Culinary Treasure

Even if turmeric isn't in your spice rack, you've probably tasted it. It's the warm, spicy, slightly bitter note in curries and many Middle Eastern dishes. Indian delicacies such as fiery hot vindaloos and tandooris benefit from its infusion of rich color and subtle but complex flavor. Even if you haven't sampled exotic cuisines, chances are you have still encountered turmeric. It's the spice that colors and lends its scent to many kinds of mustard and gives them a distinctive, vibrant golden-yellow hue. Turmeric is also a princi-

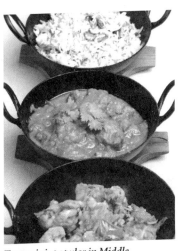

Turmeric is popular in Middle Eastern and Indian cuisine.

pal ingredient in Worcestershire sauce and is used to color and flavor butter, margarine, yellow cakes, popcorn, jellies, chutneys, relishes, seasoning blends, yogurt, cheeses, canned chicken broth, cereals, orange juice and more. Turmeric blends well with other spices, complementing chili powder, coriander, cumin and cinnamon. Like many spices, it is also a natural preservative.

Turmeric has a pungent flavor and scent. The taste of turmeric is not unlike ginger's, but sweeter and more aromatic. Some people describe it as bitter and buttery; others characterize it as peppery and earthy. Turmeric is the root of the tropical perennial known to botanists as *Curcuma longa*, a member of the *Zingiberaceae,* or ginger, family. Carolus Linnaeus (1707–1778), a Swedish botanist, classified it in 1753.

Curcuma longa is native to China but also grows in the tropical regions of India and South America. India produces nearly 90 percent of the world's supply of turmeric and is the largest producer, consumer and exporter of turmeric. Turmeric is also cultivated in Bangladesh, Thailand, Cambodia, Malaysia, Indonesia and the Philippines and also grows in parts of Africa, Brazil and the Caribbean.

Indian turmeric is considered premier and its quality is undisputed, largely because of its high curcumin content. Curcumin, the principal active constituent of turmeric, has a remarkable range of therapeutic effects, including potent antitumor, antioxidant and anti-inflammatory properties.

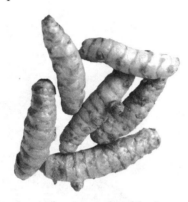

The turmeric plant is a member of the ginger family.

Curcuma longa thrives in clay-like soil in areas with high rainfall and warm temperatures. The plant grows to a height of 1 meter (approximately 3.3 feet). Its leaves are long and rectangular and its flowers are long white spikes. The plant is harvested when its leaves begin to yellow, usually about seven to nine months after planting.

Turmeric comes from the plant's rhizome—an underground horizontal stem with knobby and fingerlike branches. The rhizome is boiled and then set out to dry in the sun or in an oven, then the tough outer skins are removed, dried and ground into the rich, golden-yellow turmeric powder. Cured or processed turmeric and dried-ground turmeric are used to produce Ayurvedic medicines. (Ayurvedic medicine, or Ayurveda, is native to India and is among the oldest medicine systems in the world. In Sanskrit, *Ayurveda* means the "science of life." Some practitioners trace Ayurveda's roots back 5,000 years.)

What's in a Name?

Because of its primary active ingredient, turmeric is sometimes referred to as curcumin in the United States and other countries. According to the authors of *Turmeric: The Genus Curcuma*, the spice gets its name from the Medieval Latin term *terramerita*. Later, it became known as *terre merite* in French, which means "deserving or meritorious earth." The term *turmeric* came to us from the French language.

In ancient India, turmeric was known by many names, each describing one of its virtues, characteristics or actions:

- *Ranjani* means "that which gives color."
- *Mangal prada* and *bhadra* mean "auspicious," "lucky" or "bringing luck."
- *Krimighni* means "killing worms" and refers to turmeric's antimicrobial action.
- *Mahvigni* refers to turmeric's anti-diabetic actions.
- *Shobhna* describes turmeric's brilliant color.
- *Hemaragi* means "being the color of gold."
- *Varna-datri* means "that which gives color" and describes turmeric's use to enhance the complexion.
- *Pavitra* means "holy."
- *Haridra* shows that it is dear to Lord Krishna.
- *Anestha* means "it is not offered for sacrifice."
- *Hridayavilasani* means "delighting the heart."

In Sanskrit, turmeric has 55 synonyms that describe its medicinal or religious uses. In Hebrew, the spice is known as *kurkum*; in Spanish and Italian it is *curcuma*; and in German, *kurkuma*. In English, turmeric is sometimes called Indian saffron because turmeric and saffron share the same vibrant yellow color.

A Vivid History

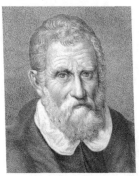

Marco Polo and other explorers introduced turmeric to Europe during the 13th century.

Even before Marco Polo described turmeric in China in 1280, the spice had been cultivated in ancient India. Some of the earliest recorded references to turmeric portray it as a remedy for jaundice and a treatment for leprosy (an infectious disease characterized by disfiguring skin sores, nerve damage and progressive debilitation).

In India, indigenous uses of turmeric in fertility rites were incorporated into Hindu ceremonies. Turmeric was associated with the fertility of the earth and the fertility of the people who inhabited it. Turmeric, which rapidly assumed an important place in Hindu traditions, was believed to have many magical qualities.

Some ancient Hindu sacred traditions endure today in India. A piece of thread, dyed yellow with turmeric, is considered auspicious and is part of Hindu wedding rituals (in other parts of the world, many people use a gold chain along with the turmeric-colored thread). In Hindu weddings, the parents of the bride and groom pour water colored with turmeric over their hands at the conclusion of the ceremony. In some areas, turmeric is painted on the doors of homes of everyone invited to a wedding. In other communities, turmeric is included, along with rice, coconuts, betel leaves, bananas, gold and silver, on a list of items that must accompany the bride to her wedding. Often newlyweds are showered with rice colored with turmeric.

There are even post-nuptial ceremonies involving turmeric. The nuptial bath involves smearing the bride with a mixture of turmeric and lime. In a ritual called *gatraharidra*, the newlywed couple is anointed with a paste made of turmeric said to enhance the libido. On the fourth day of marriage, brides paint their bodies with turmeric paste and oil and then bathe in turmeric-infused water.

Married women sometimes use turmeric to place yellow markings on their faces for special occasions, and some apply turmeric every evening. After the housework is completed, married women wash their hands in turmeric water and then touch their faces with their damp hands. Women extend this ritual to other married female visitors as well. Men also use turmeric; bridegrooms apply turmeric to their bodies to ensure good fortune, prosperity and fertility. Newborns may be fed a mixture of turmeric and coconut milk.

The ritual cosmetic use of turmeric persisted in India until the middle of the twentieth century. Turmeric also was widely used in India to dye clothes yellow, which was a popular practice because it was the color favored and worn by Lord Krishna and the Indian saint, sage and social reformer Narayana Guru (1855–1928).

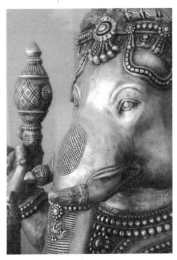

Turmeric stems are used in Ayurvedic medicine.

Turmeric also played a role in death rites. In medieval times in India, the body of a married woman who performed *sati*—burning herself in her husband's funeral pyre—was clothed in a robe colored yellow with turmeric. Applying a dusting of turmeric over the body of a person who had died became customary and was intended to purify and cleanse the body.

Turmeric was so central to Indian culture that people worshipped an icon called Turmeric Ganesha, which often takes the form of a turmeric rhizome. A turmeric and limewater mixture is still used in worship in many temples. Some historians believe that because of its brilliant yellow color, turmeric was associated with the sun and sun worship.

Turmeric most likely arrived in India from the region that today is Vietnam. It was probably transported by ancient tribal people migrating to India or by Buddhist monks traveling to India. Those travelers carried turmeric rhizomes to treat wounds and digestive disorders, which are among the same disorders turmeric is used to treat today.

Turmeric made its way into foods both as a preservative and a coloring agent, imparting a warm, appetizing deep orange or yellow hue to rice, other grains, meat and vegetables. It was likely preferred over many other members of the *Zingiberaceae* family because it was less bitter.

Turmeric's ability to treat disease was recognized early. Turmeric paste and ash from the rhizome were applied to smallpox and chicken pox lesions to help them to heal. Because of turmeric's antiseptic actions, patients were often smeared with turmeric paste and bathed in turmeric water.

The first reports of turmeric cultivation are from the Harappan civilization (in present-day Pakistan) in 3000 BCE. The techniques for cultivating, harvesting and processing turmeric are similar from one region to another and have not changed significantly over time.

Favoring Curry

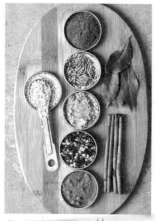

Turmeric is typically used in curry blends.

Some people mistakenly believe that curry is a spice. Although a yellow powder labeled curry is available at most supermarkets, curry is not a single spice—it's a blend of several spices. Curry varies from region to region and even from chef to chef. Not all curries are spicy hot; many are a mild, subtle blends of spices.

Indian curries generally include a basic blend of coriander, cumin, cardamom and turmeric. Other ingredients such as garlic, ginger, onions, lemon grass, cinnamon, pepper, yogurt, cream, coconut milk, ground nuts and mustard seeds may be added, depending on the recipe. Some curries include another popular northern Indian spice blend called garam masala, which may include as many as 30 ingredients, including bay leaves, black pepper, cinnamon, cloves, coriander seeds, dried chilies, fennel, mace and nutmeg.

The ingredients in curry vary to suit local palates. People in Sri Lanka toast whole spices to use in black curries. In the French West Indies, locals add mace and nutmeg to curry. In Japan, curry is sold in cubes or blocks and is compounded with spices, animal fat and fruit paste. Japanese curry is not as spicy as Indian and Thai curries and usually has a hint of sweetness not found in other curries. Thai curries are rich and creamy and often contain coconut milk and lemongrass.

Throughout the United Kingdom and much of the United States, the term *curry* refers to practically any spicy, savory Indian dish containing some combination of meat, fish and vegetables. There also are Thai and Pakistani curries, and dishes in other Asian cuisines that incorporate the traditional spice blend known as curry. But in India today, curry means sauce or gravy or a spicy stew made with a sauce as its base.

There are various explanations for the origin of the word curry. Some historians suggest it is a variation of *karil*, a term the Portuguese explorers learned in south India. Others assert that it is an Anglicized version of the Tamil word *kari*, which means "spicy sauce" and was also the name given to a south Indian soup that was served with rice. The word *curry* also may have been derived from *karahi*, a metal vessel resembling a wok that is used in Indian cooking. Alternatively, the word may have come from the similar sounding *kadhi* and *khari*, which are the names of a popular yogurt-based curry dish in northern Indian cuisine.

Incidentally, the expression "to curry favor" has nothing at all to do with the delicious spice blend. It means "to gain advancement" or "to ingratiate oneself by fawning or using insincere flattery or obsequious behavior." The expression comes from the old French words *correier*, meaning "to put in order, prepare," and *fauvel*, "the fawn colored horse." Around 1400 the phrase came into English as "curry favel" Nearly a century later it morphed into the expression used today.

The Golden Spice

Ayurvedic medicine, or Ayurveda, originated in India thousands of years ago and has been the country's primary system of medical care. Much of it is based on precepts from Hinduism, one of the oldest and most widely practiced religions in the world. The philosophical foundation for Ayurvedic medicine posits that people, their health and the universe are all intimately related. Health problems result when these complex relationships are not in balance. Imbalances—physical, emotional and spiritual—are thought to increase susceptibility to disease, and disease results from a disruption of the processes of life.

According to the National Center for Complementary and Alternative Medicine (NCCAM), which is one of the National Institutes of Heath, Ayurvedic medicine

- aims to integrate and balance the body, mind, and spirit and thereby help prevent illness and promote physical, emotional and spiritual wellness, and
- uses a variety of techniques and practices such as herbs, metals and massage to cleanse the body and restore balance.

In Ayurveda, the constitution — called the *prakriti* —is believed to be influenced by physical and psychological characteristics such as how the body uses nutrients and how it responds to stress.

The three *doshas* are important physiological principles that govern the activities of the body and interact to create health. Doshas are vital bioenergies that are known by their Sanskrit names—vata, pitta and kapha. Each dosha is composed of one or two of the five basic elements—space, air, fire, water and earth—and each is related to specific physiological functions.

Every individual has a unique balance of the three doshas, with one dosha usually being dominant. Doshas are associated with specific body types, personalities, dispositions and risks of certain health problems. Lifestyle, diet, stress and toxins may cause imbalances in a dosha.

Unlike conventional Western medicine, Ayurvedic medicine does not draw sharp distinctions between food and medicine. Overall diet and specific foods are vital aspects of Ayurvedic therapies, and herbs, plants, oils and spices (especially turmeric) are part of the Ayurvedic pharmacopeia.

In Ayurvedic medicine, turmeric is used to relieve pain, regulate menstruation, expel phlegm, aid digestion and support healthy liver function. Doses of one-half to one gram of turmeric are given for digestive disorders such as flatulence. For people with colds, coughs and congestion, inhaling the fumes of burning turmeric may stimulate the flow of mucus and immediately relieve congestion. A blend of turmeric, milk and sugar is also suggested to relieve cold symptoms.

Ayurvedic practitioners apply a paste made of turmeric directly to the skin to promote wound healing and to clear skin conditions, including eczema (characterized by redness and itchy, scaly patches). Ayurveda also employs turmeric to purify the body and mind.

Traditional Chinese Medicine

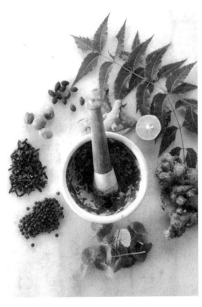

In Chinese medicine, turmeric helps balance a person's yin and yang.

Turmeric also has a long history of use in traditional Chinese medicine (TCM), another time-honored medical system. TCM has been practiced since 200 BCE. Its philosophy suggests that the body balances two opposing and connected forces: *yin* and *yang*. Optimal health arises from a balance of yin, which is cool, dark and feminine and yang, which is characterized as bright, warm and masculine.

An imbalance between yin and yang is said to block the flow of *qi* (also known as *chi*), which is the vital energy or life force, and blood along pathways through the body known as meridians. The NCCAM explains that TCM aims to restore and maintain health by bringing the body into a balanced state. TCM practitioners use a combination of herbs, acupuncture and other forms of bodywork to help unblock qi in an effort to restore harmony and wellness.

In TCM, turmeric is referred to as *jiang huang*. In Ayurveda, it is called by its Sanskrit name, *haridra*. Both traditions use turmeric to clear the channels and move the qi. Modern Western medical research has identified the potent anti-inflammatory compounds present in turmeric.

Both *Pharmacology and Applications of Chinese Materia Medica* and *Chinese Herbal Medicine Materia Medica* report that in laboratory and animal studies, turmeric has been shown to:

- reduce blood lipid levels
- improve blood circulation
- lower blood pressure
- reduce platelet aggregation (clustering or clumping of disks found in the blood that facilitate coagulation)
- promote fibrinolysis (the dissolution of clots)
- increase bile formation and secretion
- reduce inflammation
- alleviate pain
- stimulate uterine contractions

The turmeric rhizome has been used orally (alone or as part of a formula) to treat a wide range of conditions, including the following:

- digestive disorders such as dyspepsia, flatulence, abdominal bloating, abdominal pains, feelings of fullness after meals, diarrhea and loss of appetite
- parasitic infections
- hemorrhage
- hepatitis and jaundice
- liver and gallbladder complaints
- headaches
- yeast infections and fever
- amenorrhea (the absence of menstruation)
- colorectal cancer

Turmeric is applied topically as an analgesic to relieve pain and to treat ringworm, bruising, leech bites, eye infections, inflammatory skin conditions, inflammation of the mouth, swollen and painful joints and infected wounds. In Chinese folk medicine, turmeric has been used to treat digestive disorders, intermittent fevers, edema (swelling), bronchitis, colds, worms, leprosy, kidney inflammation and cystitis. Turmeric has even been used as an anticancer treatment. Turmeric is used in combination with mustard oil to treat shingles, an acute, often painful infection caused by the herpes zoster virus, the same virus that causes chicken pox. A turmeric paste may be applied to chicken pox and other lesions to help them to heal.

In TCM, turmeric is used to regulate qi, cool the blood, clear heat and ease gallbladder function. Turmeric is described as an herb that helps to invigorate and move the blood, dispelling stasis. It is termed a "digestive bitter" that helps stop the formation of intestinal gas and expel gas that has already formed. Turmeric is also a cholagogue—an agent that stimulates bile production in the liver and bile excretion via the gallbladder into the intestines. This action supports fat digestion.

TCM uses turmeric to treat congestion and chronic digestive problems such as constipation and diarrhea. Turmeric helps to relieve inflammation throughout the digestive tract and reduces spasms and cramping. Some of the digestive disorders that TCM practitioners believe may benefit from regular use of turmeric include the following:

- **Irritable bowel syndrome (IBS)**. IBS is not a single disease. It is a functional digestive disorder in which the bowel doesn't work properly. It is a syndrome, which means it is a constellation of symptoms, including abdominal pain or discomfort (cramping, bloating, gas, diarrhea or constipation). IBS affects the colon, or large intestine, the part of the digestive tract that stores fecal matter.
- **Colitis.** Colitis is inflammation of the colon that often leads to abdominal pain, fever and diarrhea with blood and mucus.
- **Crohn's disease.** Crohn's disease, also known as ileitis or enteritis, is an inflammation of the digestive tract that usually affects the ileum, the lower part of the small intestine. The inflammation and swelling can cause chronic, severe pain and diarrhea.

TCM practitioners also recommend turmeric to help restore the friendly flora (bacteria) that line the digestive tract. Those beneficial bacteria are vital for healthy digestion and immune function and must be replenished following antibiotic treatments, which can sharply reduce their ranks.

Deficiencies or imbalances in healthy intestinal flora may also lead to an overgrowth of fungi (such as *Candida albicans*) or harmful bacteria. When disease-causing bacteria predominate in the intestinal flora, their enzymes compromise digestion and the integrity of the lining of the digestive tract. Turmeric is also used to relieve itching and reduce inflammation that accompanies hemorrhoids and anal fissures.

In Chinese medicine, turmeric is also used in combination with acupuncture to relieve the symptoms of arthritis and pains in the neck, shoulders and upper back. It is also used to treat precancerous skin conditions.

In 1971, Western medicine "rediscovered" turmeric in response to reports from Indian researchers suggesting that the herb possessed anti-inflammatory and antioxidant properties. Since then, a growing body of scientific and medical literature has shown that turmeric also possesses antispasmodic, antibacterial, wound-healing and antitumor activity.

Active Ingredients

The primary chemical constituents of turmeric are curcumin, essential oils, valepotriates, alkaloids and protein. The principal active constituent of turmeric is curcumin, which makes up 2 to 5 percent of the spice. Curcumin has been the subject of numerous laboratory and animal studies that have demonstrated its various healing properties. Some research has shown curcumin to stimulate the production of bile and facilitate the emptying of the gallbladder. Curcumin has also demonstrated a protective effect on the liver, antitumor action, and an ability to reduce inflammation and fight certain kinds of infections—possibly even serious bacterial and viral infections.

Curcumin is a curcuminoid (phenolic compound). Curcuminoids were initially isolated in 1815. The chemical structure of curcumin ($C21H20O6$) was first described and synthesized in 1910 by Polish chemist Victor Lampe. Curcuminoids give turmeric its characteristic yellow color.

The figure below displays the balanced, symmetrical form of the chemical compound curcumin.

Nutrient Information

Turmeric is a good source of vitamin C and magnesium, and a very good source of dietary fiber, vitamin B6, iron and potassium. Acording to the USDA Nutrient Database, one teaspoon of ground turmeric (*Curcuma longa* L.) contains the following nutrients:

NUTRIENTS	UNIT	1.00 X 1 TSP 2.2G
Proximates		
Water	g	0.25
Energy	kcal	8
Energy	kj	33
Protein	g	0.17
Total lipid (fat)	g	0.22
Ash	g	0.13
Carbohydrate, by difference	g	1.43
Fiber, total dietary	g	0.5
Sugars, total	g	0.07
Sucrose	g	0.05
Glucose (dextrose)	g	0.01
Fructose	g	0.01
MINERALS		
Calcium, Ca	mg	4
Iron, Fe	mg	0.91
Magnesium, Mg	mg	4
Phosphorus, P	mg	6
Potassium, K	mg	56
Sodium, Na	mg	1
Zinc, Zn	mg	0.1
Copper, Cu	mg	0.013
Selenium, Se	mcg	0.1
VITAMINS		
Vitamin C, total ascorbic acid	mg	0.6
Riboflavin	mg	0.005
Niacin	mg	0.11
Vitamin B-6	mg	0.04
Folate, total	mcg	1
Folate, food	mcg	1
Folate, DFE	mcg_DFE	1
Choline, total	mg	1.1
Betaine	mg	0.2
Vitamin E (alpha-tocopherol)	mg	0.07
Tocopherol, gamma	mg	0.01
Vitamin K (phylloquinone)	mcg	0.3
LIPIDS		
Phytosterols	mg	2

USDA National Nutrient Database for Standard Reference, Release 20 (2007)

The Root of Medicine

Turmeric may very well be the most researched spice in terms of medicinal and health-promoting applications. Because curcumin has been shown to have antioxidant, anti-inflammatory, antiviral, antibacterial, antifungal and anticancer actions, it has the potential to address a wide range of diseases, including diabetes, allergies, arthritis, Alzheimer's disease and other chronic diseases.

Laboratory cell culture and animal studies suggest that curcumin has tremendous potential as an antiproliferative, anti-invasive and antiangiogenic agent; as a mediator of chemoresistance (protecting against damage from chemicals or drugs and the effects of drugs) and radioresistance (helping to protect against damage caused by radiation); as a chemopreventive agent to protect against the development of a wide range of diseases; and as a therapeutic agent in wound healing, diabetes, Alzheimer's disease, Parkinson's disease, cardiovascular disease, pulmonary disease and arthritis.

These actions are mediated through the regulation of various transcription factors, growth factors, inflammatory cytokines, protein kinases and other enzymes. Curcumin has demonstrated actions comparable to drugs that block tumor necrosis (death of living tissue).

Anti-Inflammatory Actions

Traditionally known for its powerful anti-inflammatory action, curcumin has the potential to treat a wide variety of inflammatory diseases, including cancer, diabetes, cardiovascular disease, arthritis, Alzheimer's disease, psoriasis and more.

In order to understand curcumin's anti-inflammatory effects, it's important to understand the inflammatory process. Inflammation is the activation of the immune system response to infection, irritation or injury. An inflammatory response entails an influx of white blood cells, redness, heat, swelling, pain and dysfunction of the organs involved. Inflammation is a healthy first response to infections and wounds.

However, when inflammation persists, the immune system remains in a chronic state of high alert. This forces the body to produce high levels of specialized immune system chemicals called cytokines and gives rise to energy-robbing oxidative stress that may, in turn, lead to chronic disease.

The suffix —*itis* means inflammation and is applied to various body parts and organs: arthritis is inflammation of the joints, rhinitis is inflammation of the nose, cystitis is inflammation of the bladder and sinusitis is inflammation of the sinuses. Inflammation is also involved in a variety of "non-itis" diseases such as allergies, asthma, diabetes, heart disease, irritable bowel syndrome and many cancers.

The anti-inflammatory activity of turmeric has been demonstrated and confirmed in laboratory studies and animal models. When administered by injection in the laboratory, its effectiveness is reportedly similar to that of hydrocortisone acetate (the active ingredient in many over-the-counter and prescription creams used to reduce itching, redness, and swelling associated with many skin conditions), phenylbutazone (a non-steroidal anti-inflammatory drug used to treat chronic pain, including the symptoms of arthritis) and indomethacin (a non-steroidal anti-inflammatory drug commonly used to reduce fever, pain, stiffness and swelling).

Curcumin's advantage over some pharmaceutical anti-inflammatories is that it has a long history of safety and is inexpensive and well tolerated. There have been no serious side effects and no toxicity reported with its use. In contrast, many anti-inflammatory drugs have the potential to produce serious side effects.

The anti-inflammatory activity of curcumin may involve the inhibition of two enzymes: trypsin, which breaks down proteins, and hyaluronidase, which breaks down carbohydrate molecules called proteoglycans. Curcumin binds to a variety of proteins and inhibits the activity of various kinases. Its ability to scavenge oxygen radicals, which have been implicated in the inflammation process, may also explain some of curcumin's actions.

Curcumin regulates the expression of inflammatory enzymes, cytokines, adhesion molecules and cell survival proteins. Curcumin also affects the nuclear transcription factor kappa-B (NF-κB), a protein complex involved in the immune response to infection and inflammatory reactions. NF-κB contributes to such diseases as rheumatoid arthritis, asthma and cancer.

Curcumin or "Curecumin"?

Based on curcumin's excellent safety profile and multiple therapeutic actions, investigators at Baylor University Medical Center in Texas, wrote in the February 2008 issue of *Biochemical Pharmacology* that, "A spice once relegated to the kitchen shelf, has moved into the clinic and may prove to be 'curecumin.'" Past trials indicate a potential therapeutic role for curcumin in diseases such as familial adenomatous polyposis (an inherited condition in which numerous polyps form in the colon and rectum), inflammatory bowel disease, ulcerative colitis, colon cancer, pancreatic cancer, hypercholesteremia (high cholesterol levels), atherosclerosis, pancreatitis, psoriasis, chronic anterior uveitis (inflammation of the uveal tract, the pigmented layers of the eye) and arthritis.

If, after the completion of the many clinical trials currently underway in the United States, Europe and Asia, curcumin proves to be as effective as preliminary research suggests, it will not be the first time a naturally occurring substance becomes a widely used therapeutic agent. Aspirin was derived from willow bark. Digitalis, which is used to treat several heart conditions, is made from the leaves of the foxglove plant. And artemisinin, which is used to treat malaria, came from a shrub used in TCM.

Relief for Arthritis?

The word *arthritis* literally means joint inflammation and refers to more than 100 related conditions and disorders known as rheumatic diseases. When a joint becomes inflamed, swelling, redness, pain and loss of motion occur. In the most serious cases, the loss of motion can be disabling.

Most instances of inflammation are normal, healthy responses to an injury or a disease. Inflammation causes pain, redness, swelling and warmth in the affected body part. Once the injury is healed or the disease is cured, the inflammation stops. In arthritis, however, the inflammation does not subside. Instead, it becomes part of the problem, damaging healthy tissues and generating more inflammation and more damage as the painful cycle continues. The damage can change the shape of bones and other tissues of the joints, making movement difficult and painful.

Turmeric and curcumin are ingredients in many supplements formulated to help relieve arthritis pain and inflammation. Curcumin, the active ingredient in turmeric, has powerful anti-inflammatory and antioxidant components and may treat the joint inflammation, stiffness and swelling resulting from arthritis.

Multiple laboratory studies have confirmed turmeric's antiinflammatory and antiarthritic activity. The first such study was a small double-blind study published in 1980 in the *Indian Journal of Medical Research*. In this study, researchers gave patients with rheumatoid arthritis curcumin (1,200 mg/day) or a non-steroidal anti-inflammatory drug, phenylbutazine (300 mg/day). The patients taking curcumin reported and were observed to have significant improvements (compared to the group treated with phenylbutazine) in terms of morning stiffness, walking time and joint swelling. The improvements were noted after just two weeks of taking curcumin.

In 2006, researchers from the University of Arizona compared the chemical composition of an experimental turmeric extract with over-the-counter turmeric supplements. The researchers studied the influence of the experimental turmeric extract on joint inflammation and destruction and its effect on genetic markers associated with inflammation. They also explored turmeric's mechanism of action in an effort to pinpoint exactly how it protects against joint inflammation.

The researchers found that a turmeric extract with curcumin appeared to be effective at blocking rheumatoid arthritis in rats by preventing NF-κB activation in the joints. The turmeric extract also blocked a pathway associated with bone loss, indicating that turmeric may benefit people with osteoporosis (loss of bone mass and density).

The researchers also discovered that non-curcumin components of turmeric are anti-inflammatory. These components may act synergistically with one another and with curcumin to block inflammation. The researchers concluded that "Just as the willow bark provided relief for arthritis patients before the advent of aspirin, it would appear that the underground stem (rhizome) of a tropical plant may also hold promise for the treatment of joint inflammation and destruction."

In 2008, researchers in Israel reported that adding curcumin, a natural COX-2 inhibitor (non-steroidal anti inflammatory drug), to a treatment regimen using a prescription COX-2-specific inhibitor synergistically augmented the effects of the drug in laboratory and animal models up to a staggering 1,000 percent. That action resulted in a drug efficacy at a markedly lower dose—up to 10 times lower than drug-produced therapeutic effects. These and other promising findings have prompted scientists to posit that turmeric may be helpful for other inflammatory conditions such as carpal tunnel syndrome, joint inflammation and post-workout muscle inflammation.

Skin Diseases and Wound Healing

Curcumin has been used to prevent and treat skin diseases and skin complications of diseases such as scleroderma, psoriasis and skin cancer. Curcumin is thought to protect skin by reducing free radicals and inflammation by inhibiting NF-κB.

Wound healing involves a systematic progression of events that reestablish the integrity of damaged tissue. Curcumin speeds wound healing by inducing transforming growth factor-beta, which promotes angiogenesis and the growth of extracellular matrix. It also improves collagen synthesis and deposition and increases the density of blood vessels.

In 2005, researchers found that a pretreatment with curcumin helped to heal radiation-induced skin injuries such as those that may occur as a result of radiation therapy. Radiation disrupts normal responses to injury, leading to a prolonged recovery period. Curcumin pretreatment significantly increased the rate of wound contraction and decreased wound healing time. It also enhanced many aspects of the wound healing process, including the synthesis of collagen, hexosamine, DNA, nitrite and improved collagen deposition and vascular density.

In 2006, investigators at the University of North Carolina, Chapel Hill, observed the effects of topical administration of curcumin on the collagen characteristics and antioxidant properties of skin during wound healing. Curcumin increased cellular proliferation and collagen synthesis at the wound site. It also decreased the oxidative degradation of lipids (fat soluble molecules) and increased the activity of enzymes that accelerate would healing. The investigators concluded that, overall, curcumin hastened healing.

These studies hint at curcumin's beneficial effects and potential to be developed as a potent, natural, nontoxic agent for treating skin diseases.

Preventing Cataracts

A cataract is a clouding of the naturally clear lens of the eye. The prevalence of cataracts increases dramatically with age. Most cataracts develop slowly but progress over time, causing cloudy vision and, eventually, almost complete blindness. Once a cataract develops, surgically removing the affected lens and replacing it with an artificial lens is the only treatment currently available.

Each year about 1.5 million cataract surgeries are performed, making cataract surgury the most common surgical procedure in the United States for people over age 65. Scientists estimate that delaying the development of cataracts by 10 years could reduce the need for cataract surgery by as much as half. According to the National Eye Institute, more than half of all Americans have cataracts by age 80. People with diabetes have an increased risk of developing cataracts.

Oxidative stress may be the underlying mechanism responsible for the development of cataracts. Heightening the antioxidant defenses of the ocular lens has been shown to prevent or delay the development of cataracts. Curcumin may protect against cataract formation induced by the oxidative degeneration of lipids.

Any strategy that prevents or slows the progression of cataracts has a significant impact on the health of aging populations. Animal studies suggest that turmeric and curcumin can help to delay the development and progression of cataracts.

Inflammatory Bowel Disease

Inflammatory bowel disease (IBD) is a chronic inflammation of the intestinal tract. IBD includes two different conditions: ulcerative colitis, in which sores or ulcers form in the innermost layers of the lining of the large intestine, and Crohn's disease, which also causes inflammation of the digestive tract.

Crohn's disease can affect any part of the digestive tract but most often affects the ileum, the lower part of the small intestine. The swelling extends deep into the lining of the affected organ. In general, Crohn's disease tends to be more severe than ulcerative colitis, though both are serious and debilitating for many sufferers.

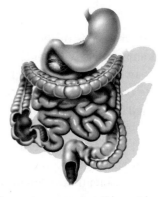

Curcumin can ease the inflammation associated with IBS.

Symptoms of ulcerative colitis and Crohn's disease are similar and include abdominal pain, cramps and loose discharges of pus, blood and mucus from the bowel. There are three possible, but as yet unproven causes of IBD. The first is persistent infection with a specific agent, though none have been identified or isolated. The second is a defective mucosal barrier. The third is an overly aggressive immune response. Recent genetic and genomics research has identified multiple genes linked to Crohn's disease and ulcerative colitis. The interactions of these genes with one another and with environmental risk factors such as smoking may explain the development of some cases of IBD.

A number of therapies that have been used to treat IBD target the transcription factor NF-κB, which is involved in inflammation. In 2003, investigators in Vancouver found that curcumin was able to significantly ease and reduce inflammation in IBD. Although it is not known precisely how curcumin accomplished that, the investigators speculate that curcumin's effects on the immune system likely rely on curcumin's antioxidant properties, activation of NF-κB and ability to reduce the expression of proinflammatory cytokines.

Since 2003, researchers have amassed evidence that curcumin modulates the immune system and disrupts the proinflammatory cascade through a variety of mechanisms, including antioxidant effects, alterations in cell signaling and disruption of bacterial flora. Curcumin also may help to relieve symptoms of IBD by inhibiting the growth of new blood vessels in the intestines, COX-2 (an enzyme involved in inflammation) expression and prostanoid production.

Alzheimer's Disease

Alzheimer's disease (AD) is a progressive degenerative disease that affects the brain and results in severely impaired memory, thinking and behavior. It is a disease, not a normal consequence of aging. The NIH reports that AD is the seventh leading cause of death in the United States. Even though nearly three-quarters of AD sufferers are older than 70, the disease can strike people as early as their thirties, forties and fifties.

A German physician, Alois Alzheimer (1864–1915), first described the disease in 1907 after he had cared for a patient with an unusual mental illness. Alzheimer observed changes in his patient's brain and described them as abnormal clumps and tangled bundles of fibers. Nearly a century later, those abnormal clumps, along with abnormal clusters of proteins in the brain, are recognized as the hallmarks of AD. Inflammation of the brain is also associated with AD.

AD begins slowly. Its symptoms include cognitive decline and impaired memory, speech loss and personality changes. AD sufferers may also experience confusion; language problems such as trouble finding words; impaired judgment; temporal and spatial disorientation; and changes in mood, behavior and personality. Because there is no cure for AD, treatment focuses on managing symptoms.

Although several genes are linked to its development, to date there has been no way to prevent AD. A number of studies suggest that turmeric may hold a key to preventing and treating AD and other neurodegenerative diseases. As is the case in many other diseases, oxidative stress has been implicated in nerve cell injury in AD and other neurological diseases.

Alzheimer's disease involves a chronic inflammatory respone associated with both brain injury and beta-amyloid (insoluble fibrous proteins in the brain) dysfunction There is mounting evidence that factors such as oxidative stress, disturbed protein metabolism and their interaction are fundamental in the development and progression of AD. Curcumin has been considered as a nutritional approach to reduce oxidative damage and the amyloid disorder associated with AD.

Population studies find that India, where turmeric consumption is frequent and widespread, has one of the lowest rates of AD anywhere in the world. Although there are many possible explanations for the low rate of AD, it is possible that routine consumption of turmeric helps to prevent the disease.

Animal studies confirm that curcumin affects oxidation, inflammation and cholesterol—all of which are believed to be important in the development of AD. Furthermore, animal studies point to a direct effect of curcumin in decreasing the amyloid involved in AD. In more than one study, mice fed low doses of curcumin had significantly reduced levels of amyloid plaque. Curcumin has also been found to cross the blood-brain barrier in mice and is therefore able to directly bind to amyloid plaques.

Researchers are trying to pinpoint how curcumin prevents and slows the progression of AD in animals. Investigators in China think curcumin may chelate metal, reducing amyloid or oxidative toxicity to the nerve cells. These investigators found that curcumin binds iron and copper, and they hypothesize that curcumin protects against amyloid aggregation or suppresses inflammatory damage by preventing metal induction of NF-κB.

Research conducted in Singapore found that older adults who reported frequent, or at least occasional, consumption of curry fared better on the Mini-Mental State Examination (MMSE) cognitive test than those who never consumed curry. This finding led the investigators to hypothesize that diets supplemented with curry benefit cognitive function. In the United States, clinical trials are under way to determine whether curcumin can prevent the buildup of amyloid plaques that characterize the brains of Alzheimer's patients.

Protection Against Brain Injury

The neuroprotective role of curcumin that has been demonstrated in laboratory and animal studies is largely attributed to the antioxidant and anti-inflammatory effects of curcumin.

Researchers have found that curcumin can protect the brain from injury. In one animal study in which blood supply to the brain was cut off, animals treated with curcumin fared better in terms of damage to the brain and resulting sensory motor function losses than animals that had not been given curcumin.

Another animal study found that curcumin possesses anticonvulsant activity and was also able to reduce seizure activity, which means it may have the potential to help people suffering from seizure disorders such as epilepsy.

Curcumin offers at least 10 known neuroprotective actions. Many of these may be developed as therapies for major disabling age-related neurodegenerative diseases, such as Parkinson's disease and stroke, and diseases that result from immune dysfunction, such as multiple sclerosis and myasthenia gravis.

Heart Disease

Alzheimer's disease and cardiovascular disease are chronic diseases associated with aging that share certain characteristics and risk factors involving lipoproteins, oxidative damage and inflammation. Curcumin has demonstrated many actions that may help to protect against these shared characteristics.

Heart disease is the leading cause of death in the United States. The Centers for Disease Control and Prevention report that about 700,000 people die of heart disease in the United States each year and that nearly 30 percent of all deaths are attributable to heart disease. An estimated 14 million people in the United States suffer from coronary heart disease (also called coronary artery disease), which is the most common type of heart disease.

The most common cause of coronary heart disease is an accumulation of plaque—a combination of fatty material, calcium and scar tissue—in the coronary arteries that supply the heart with blood, oxygen and other nutrients. The coronary arteries are strong and flexible, and in healthy young people their linings are smooth and allow for unobstructed blood flow.

With advancing age, deposits of plaque cause the arteries to thicken and become less elastic. Atherosclerosis, or hardening of the arteries, describes the condition when there is enough plaque to obstruct the flow of blood. Artherosclerosis causes ischemia, or inadequate blood supply. Plaque deposits in the coronary arteries not only restrict blood flow to the heart but can also become dislodged and promote blood clotting.

Curcumin may help to inhibit atherosclerosis, in part by preventing the oxidation of cholesterol. Ideally, total cholesterol as measured in the blood should be 200 or less. Low-density lipoprotein (LDL is the "bad" cholesterol associated with increased risk for heart disease) should be less than 100, and high-density lipoprotein (HDL is the "good" cholesterol associated with reduced risk for heart disease) should be 60 or higher. In addition to lowering blood cholesterol and preventing LDL oxidation, research reveals that curcumin inhibits platelet aggregation, prevents thrombosis and helps to limit damage to the heart muscle if its blood supply is transiently reduced.

Cancer

Cancer is a large group of diseases characterized by the uncontrolled growth and spread of abnormal cells. Those cells may grow into masses of tissue called tumors. Non-cancerous tumors are benign tumors. Cancerous tumors are malignant tumors. The danger of cancer is that cancer cells invade and destroy normal tissue.

One of the most exciting findings about curcumin is its potential to prevent and treat various forms of cancer. Carcinogenesis, the development of cancer, involves three stages: initiation, progression and promotion. Curcumin appears to be beneficial in inhibiting all three stages of carcinogenesis. Its anticancer actions may be due to its inhibition of NF-κB and subsequent inhibition of proinflammatory pathways as well as its ability to prevent the growth of new blood vessels.

One approach to reducing the prevalence of cancer is to use chemopreventive agents—safe compounds that protect against the development of cancer. Curcumin may have a role in the prevention of colon cancer and other cancers. Investigators at the University of Texas Medical Branch at Galveston have found that curcumin blocked the activity of neurotensin, a hormone involved in the development of colon cancer. Although curcumin is poorly absorbed after ingestion, many studies suggest that even low doses of curcumin may be sufficient for its chemopreventive and chemotherapeutic activity.

Curcumin's potent antioxidant action protects cells from the free radicals that can harm cellular DNA. This is especially important in cells that undergo frequent turnover, such as those that line the digestive tract, because when these cells become cancerous they can reproduce quickly.

Clinical trials have demonstrated that curcumin is well tolerated and safe, and many studies suggest that it is effective. Curcumin has been shown to inhibit the proliferation of various tumor cells in cell cultures, to prevent carcinogen-induced cancers in rodents, and to inhibit the growth of tumors in animal models, either alone or in combination with chemotherapeutic drugs or radiation. Other clinical trials suggest that curcumin exerts antitumor effects in people with precancerous lesions or people who are at a high risk of developing cancer.

In the laboratory, curcumin has demonstrated anticancer effects on breast cancer tumor cells, as well as on colon cancer, stomach cancer, kidney cancer, liver cancer, ovarian cancer and lung cancer. It has also been shown to inhibit the proliferation of leukemia. Animal studies report that curcumin inhibited tumor promotion in skin and prevented the development of breast cancer, oral cancer, stomach cancer, liver cancer, prostate cancer and colon cancer.

In 2006, investigators at Johns Hopkins University and the Cleveland Clinic reported that a combination of curcumin and quercetin reduced the size and number of precancerous lesions in patients with colorectal polyps. The same year, investigators in Israel reported that curcumin inhibited growth of malignant pancreatic and lung cells by down-regulating COX-2 activity and epidermal growth factor receptor (EGFR). EGFR is the protein found on the surface of some cells and to which epidermal growth factor binds, causing the cells to divide. EGFR is found at abnormally high levels on the surface of many types of cancer cells, so those cells may divide excessively in the presence of epidermal growth factor.

In 2007, researchers reported that curcumin reduced prostate cancer cell production of MDM2, a protein involved in the formation of cancerous tumors. Curcumin also spurred cells to produce another protein associated with apoptosis (programmed cell death) and inhibited cancer cell proliferation. In 2008, investigators in Thailand described the process by which curcumin prevents metastasis, the spread of cancer cells throughout the body.

Curcumin has also been shown to enhance the efficacy of chemotherapeutic agents such as gemcitabine, used to treat pancreatic cancer, and oxaliplatin, used to treat colon cancer. Curcumin prevents tumor cells from becoming resistant to drugs and also boosts the effectiveness of some cancer drugs.

One of the leading proponents of curcumin as a cancer treatment is Bharat Aggarwal, a scientist at the University of Texas M. D. Anderson Cancer Center. Aggarwal, who has been researching the anticancer activity of the spice for nearly three decades, opines that curcumin is a vital cancer treatment because it regulates multiple targets—down-regulating some and up-regulating others—which is needed for the treatment of most diseases. He also observes that curcumin is inexpensive and has been found to be safe in human clinical trials.

Asserting that cancer is largely a disease of old age, and observing curcumin's ability to combat leukemia, lymphoma, gastrointestinal cancers, genitourinary cancers, breast cancer, ovarian cancer, head and neck squamous cell carcinoma, lung cancer, melanoma, neurological cancers and sarcoma, Aggarwal concludes that "An 'old-age' disease such as cancer requires an 'age-old' treatment."

Cystic Fibrosis

Cystic fibrosis (CF) is the most common inherited fatal disease in children and young adults in the United States. CF occurs in about one of 3,200 Caucasians, one of 15,000 African Americans, and one of 31,000 Asian Americans. CF causes a relatively modest impairment of chloride transport in cells. Chloride is one of the most important minerals in the blood—it helps keep the amount of fluid inside and outside of cells in balance—and the seemingly minor defect in chloride transport can result in a multi-system disease that provokes abnormal, thick secretions from glands and epithelial cells. Ultimately, those secretions fill the lungs and cause people with CF to die of respiratory failure.

Researchers believe that curcumin may be useful in the treatment of degenerative diseases, including cystic fibrosis. Curcumin has been shown to correct CF caused by a mutation of the cystic fibrosis transmembrane regulator (CFTR), but exactly how it does that remains unclear. Investigators in Japan posit that curcumin down-regulates calreticulin, a protein that binds calcium ions, which in turn suppresses expression of the faulty gene.

The Cystic Fibrosis Foundation in Bethesda, Maryland, is underwriting research on a variety of therapies, including curcumin, aimed at correcting the defective CFTR protein made by the CF gene. These therapies will allow chloride and sodium to move properly in cells lining the lungs and other organs. The foundation reports that while curcumin appeared to correct the abnormal processing of CFTR in some mice, preliminary research in humans has not produced comparable results.

Fighting Infection

Curcumin may combat bacterial, viral and parasitic infections. More than a decade ago, turmeric oil and curcumin were found to be effective as topical preparations against mold and yeast. One study reported that applying turmeric oil to skin lesions produced a healing response in two to five days, and that the lesions completely disappeared in one week.

Another potential topical use of curcumin is to prevent viral infection. Curcumin has demonstrated action against herpes simplex virus type 2, a common sexually transmitted infection, and is effective against coxsackievirus, a group of viruses that produce a disease in humans characterized by fever and rash.

Curcumin has proven effective against *Helicobacter pylori*, a bacterium that can harm the lining of the stomach and upper small intestine and cause ulcers, and against *Pseudomonas aeruginosa*, a bacterium commonly isolated from wounds, burns and urinary tract infections that also is a common cause of hospital-acquired infections. Curcumin has also been found to be antimalarial. (Malaria is an infectious disease transmitted by the bite of infected mosquitoes.) Curcumin is effective against parasitic diseases as well, including *Giardia lamblia,* a major source of intestinal infections throughout the world.

Make Your Own Curry

It's easy to make a fresh blend of curry spices. For a simple curry recipe, toast coriander seeds, nutmeg, fennel seeds, cumin seeds, anise seeds, fenugreek seeds, turmeric and cayenne in either a skillet or a toaster oven. Be careful not to burn them! In a skillet, the spices will darken and become richly fragrant in less than three minutes.

The turmeric and cayenne need even less time—less than a minute of heat will bring out their aromas and flavors.

Although it's traditional to use a mortar and pestle to grind spices, it's much easier to use a clean electric coffee grinder. Grind the toasted spices—except the turmeric and cayenne— along with some green or black cardamom until the spices are a fine powder. Strain the ground spices into a bowl and mix in some turmeric and cayenne. Allow the blend to cool completely and then store it in an airtight container in a cool, dry cupboard.

For an even fresher flavor, prepare the toasted spice—two tablespoons each of cumin seeds, cardamom seeds and coriander seeds—and combine them with 1/4 cup of ground turmeric, one teaspoon of dry mustard, and one teaspoon of cayenne in a container with an airtight lid. (For a spicier, curry, add some chili powder and black peppercorns.) When you are ready to use your curry, simply grind the amount you will need for your recipe.

To make an instant curry powder that requires no toasting, baking or grinding, combine five tablespoons ground coriander seeds, two tablespoons ground cumin seeds, one tablespoon ground turmeric, two teaspoons ground ginger, two teaspoons dry mustard, two teaspoons ground fenugreek seeds, 1 1/2 teaspoons ground black pepper, one teaspoon ground cinnamon, 1/2 teaspoon ground cloves, 1/2 teaspoon ground cardamom and 1/2 teaspoon ground chili peppers.

Use curry to spice up chicken salad, deviled eggs or egg salad; to add flavor to roasted root vegetables, rice, boiled potatoes, potato salad, chickpeas or steamed cauliflower; and to flavor chicken, beef and fish.

Perhaps no other spice has such a varied place in history. Turmeric's social, dietary and medicinal uses chronicle its importance in several of the world's oldest cultures. Whether ingested or applied topically, turmeric may deliver health benefits because of its powerful anti-inflammatory, antiviral, antioxidant, antibacterial, antifungal and anticancer potential. Adding this unusual and exotic spice to the diet is a culinary adventure well worth the effort.

References

Agricultural Research Service. 2007. "Oxygen Radical Absorbance Capacity (ORAC) of selected foods—2007." United States Department of Agriculture. http://www.ars.usda. gov/SP2UserFiles/Place/12354500/Data/ORAC/ORAC07.pdf.

Ak, T. and I. Gülçin. 2008. "Antioxidant and radical scavenging properties of curcumin." *Chemico-Biological Interactions* 174(1): 27–37.

Anand, P. et al. 2008. "Curcumin and cancer: An 'old-age' disease with an 'age-old' solution." *Cancer Letters* 267(1): 133–64.

Apisariyakul, A. et al. 1995. "Antifungal activity of turmeric oil extracted from *Curcuma longa* (Zingiberaceae)." *Journal of Ethnopharmacology* 49(3): 163–69.

Awasthi, S. et al. 1996. "Curcumin protects against 4-hydroxy-2-trans-nonenal-induced cataract formation in rat lenses." *American Journal of Clinical Nutrition* 64(5): 761–66.

Baum, L. and A. Ng. 2004. "Curcumin interaction with copper and iron suggests one possible mechanism of action in Alzheimer's disease animal models." *Journal of Alzheimer's Disease* 6(4): 367–77.

Bensky, D. and A. Gamble. 1993. *Chinese Herbal Medicine: Materia Medica,* rev. ed. Seattle, WA: Eastland.

Bharal, N. et al. 2008. "Curcumin has anticonvulsant activity on increasing current electro-shock seizures in mice." *Phytotherapy Research* Jul 25 (Epub ahead of print).

Binion, D.G. et al. 2008. "Curcumin inhibits VEGF mediated angiogenesis in human intestinal microvascular endothelial cells through COX-2 and MAPK inhibition." *Gut* Jul 2 (Epub ahead of print).

Bourne, K.Z. et al. 1999. "Plant products as topical microbicide candidates: assessment of in vitro and in vivo activity against herpes simplex virus type 2." *Antiviral Research* 42(3): 219–26.

Bright, J.J. 2007. "Curcumin and autoimmune disease." *Advances in Experimental Medicine and Biology* 595:425–51.

Chandra, V. et al. 2001. "Incidence of Alzheimer's disease in a rural community in India: the Indo-US study." *Neurology* 57(6): 985–89.

Chang, H.M. and P.P.H. But, eds. 1986. *Pharmacology and Applications of Chinese Materia Medica* (2 vols.). Singapore: World Scientific.

Cystic Fibrosis Foundation. 2008. "Drug Development Pipeline." http://www.cff.org/research/DrugDevelopmentPipeline.

Deodhar, S.D. et al. 1980. "Preliminary study on antirheumatic activity of curcumin (diferuloyl methane)." *Indian Journal of Medical Research* 71.632 38

Dharmananda, S. 1999. "Turmeric: what's in an herb name? How turmeric (jianghuang) and curcuma (yujin) became confused." *Institute for Traditional Medicine.* http://www. itmonline.org/arts/turmeri3.htm.

Dickerman, S. 2002. "Curry." *Food & Wine* March.

Dohare P. et al. 2008. "Dose dependence and therapeutic window for the neuroprotective effects of curcumin in thromboembolic model of rat." *Behavioural Brain Research* 193(2): 289–97.

Foryst-Ludwig, A. et al. 2004. "Curcumin blocks NF-kappaB and the motogenic response in *Helicobacter pylori*–infected epithelial cells." *Biochemical and Biophysical Research Communications* 316(4): 1065–72.

Funk, J.L. 2006. "Efficacy and mechanism of action of turmeric supplements in the treatment of experimental arthritis." *Arthritis and Rheumitism* 54(11): 3452–64.

Goel, A. et al. 2008. "Curcumin as "curecumin": from kitchen to clinic." *Biochemical Pharmacology* 75(4): 787–809.

Goel, A. et al. 2008. "Multi-targeted therapy by curcumin: how spicy is it?" *Molecular Nutrition and Food Research* 52(9): 1010–30.

Harada, K. et al. 2007. "Curcumin enhances cystic fibrosis transmembrane regulator expression by down-regulating calreticulin." *Biochemical and Biophysical Research Communications* 353(2): 351–56.

Jagetia, G.C. and G.K. Rajanikant. 2005. "Curcumin treatment enhances the repair and regeneration of wounds in mice exposed to hemibody gamma-irradiation." *Plastic and Reconstructive Surgery* 115(2): 515–28.

Johnson, J.J. and H. Mukhtar. 2007. "Curcumin for chemoprevention of colon cancer." *Cancer Letters* 255(2): 170–81.

Kamat, A.M. et al. 2007. "Curcumin potentiates the apoptotic effects of chemotherapeutic agents and cytokines through down-regulation of nuclear factor-kappa B and nuclear factor-kappa B-regulated gene products in IFN-alpha-sensitive and IFN-alpha-resistant human bladder cancer cells." *Molecular Cancer Therapeutics* 6(3): 1022–33.

Kasinski, A.L. et al. 2008. "Inhibition of IKK-NF-[kappa]B signaling pathway by EF24, a novel monoketone analogue of curcumin." *Molecular Pharmacology Fast Forward* (June 24).

Khanna, D. et al. 2007. "Natural products as a gold mine for arthritis treatment." *Current Opinion in Pharmacology* 7(3): 344–51.

Kunnumakkara, A.B. et al. 2007. "Curcumin potentiates antitumor activity of gemcitabine in an orthotopic model of pancreatic cancer through suppression of proliferation, angiogenesis, and inhibition of nuclear factor-kappa B-regulated gene products." *Cancer Research* 67(8): 3853–61.

Kunnumakkara, A.B. et al. 2008. "Curcumin inhibits proliferation, invasion, angiogenesis and metastasis of different cancers through interaction with multiple cell signaling proteins." *Cancer Letters* 269(2): 199–225.

Lee, H.S. et al. 2007. "Neuroprotective effect of curcumin is mainly mediated by blockade of microglial cell activation." *Die Pharmazie* 62(12): 937–42.

Lev-Ari, S. et al. 2006. "Inhibition of pancreatic and lung adenocarcinoma cell survival by curcumin is associated with increased apoptosis, down-regulation of COX-2 and EGFR and inhibition of Erk1/2 activity." *Anticancer Research* 26(6B): 4423–30.

Lev-Ari, S. et al. 2008. "Compositions for treatment of cancer and inflammation." Recent Patents on Anticancer Drug Discovery 3(1): 55–62.

Li, M. et al. 2007. "Curcumin, a dietary component has antiproliferative and chemosensitization, and radiosensitization effects by regulating the MDM2 oncogene through the PI3K/mTOR/ETS2 pathway." *Cancer Research* 67(5): 1988–96.

López-Lázaro, M. 2008. "Anticancer and carcinogenic properties of curcumin: considerations for its clinical development as a cancer chemopreventive and chemotherapeutic agent." *Molecular Nutrition and Food Research* 52 (Suppl 1): S103–27.

Majeed, M. et al. 1996. *Turmeric and the Healing Curcuminoids.* New Canaan, CT: Keats.

Malhi, M. "History of curry." Hub-UK. http://www.hub-uk.com/interesting/curry-history.htm.

National Center for Complementary and Alternative Medicine. 2008. "Whole medical systems: an overview." National Institutes of Health. http://nccam.nih.gov/health/backgrounds/wholemed.htm.

National Digestive Diseases Information Clearinghouse. 2008. "Digestive diseases news spring/summer 2008: genomics research yielding personalized approach to IBD treatment." National Institute of Diabetes and Digestive and Kidney Diseases. http://

digestive.niddk.nih.gov/about/ddnews/spr08/1.htm.

Ng, T.P. et al. 2006. "Curry consumption and cognitive function in the elderly." *American Journal of Epidemiology* 164(9): 898–906.

Padmaja, S. and T.N. Raju. 2004. "Antioxidant effect of curcumin in selenium induced cataract of Wistar rats." *Indian Journal of Experimental Biology* 42(6): 601–03.

Panchatcharam, M. et al. 2006. "Curcumin improves wound healing by modulating collagen and decreasing reactive oxygen species." *Molecular and Cellular Biochemistry* 290(1–2): 87–96.

Pérez-Arriaga, L. et al. 2006. "Cytotoxic effect of curcumin on *Giardia lamblia* trophozoites." *Acta Tropica* 98(2): 152–61.

Peschel, D. et al. 2007. "Curcumin induces changes in expression of genes involved in cholesterol homeostasis." *Journal of Nutritional Biochemistry* 18(2): 113–19.

Ravindran, P.N. et al. 2007. *Turmeric: The Genus Curcuma.* Boca Raton, FL: CRC.

Reddy, R.C. et al. 2005. "Curcumin for malaria therapy." *Biochemical and Biophysical Research Communications* 326(2): 472–74.

Ringman, J.M. et al. "A potential role of the curry spice curcumin in Alzheimer's disease." *Current Alzheimer Research* 2(2): 131–36.

Rudrappa, T. and H.P. Bais. 2008. "Curcumin, a known phenolic from *Curcuma longa*, attenuates the virulence of *Pseudomonas aeruginosa* PAO1 in whole plant and animal pathogenicity models." *Journal of Agricultural and Food Chemistry* 56(6): 1955–62.

Rukkumani, R. et al. 2005. "Comparative effects of curcumin and its analog on alcohol- and polyunsaturated fatty acid–induced alterations in circulatory lipid profiles." *Journal of Medicinal Food* 8(2): 256–60.

Salh, B. et al. 2003. "Curcumin attenuates DNB-induced murine colitis." *American Journal of Physiology. Gastrointestinal and Liver Physiology* 285(1): G235–43.

Shishodia, S. et al. 2007. "Modulation of transcription factors by curcumin." *Advances in Experimental Medicine and Biology* 595:127–48.

Si, X. et al. 2007. "Dysregulation of the ubiquitin-proteasome system by curcumin suppresses coxsackievirus B3 replication." *Journal of Virology* 81(7): 3142–50.

Strimpakos, A.S. and R.A. Sharma. 2008. "Curcumin: preventive and therapeutic properties in laboratory studies and clinical trials." *Antioxidants and Redox Signaling* 10(3): 511–45.

Suryanarayana, P. et al. 2005. "Curcumin and turmeric delay streptozotocin-induced diabetic cataract in rats." *Investigative Ophthalmology and Visual Science* 46(6): 2092–99.

Thangapazham, R.L. et al. 2006. "Multiple molecular targets in cancer chemoprevention by curcumin." *AAPS Journal* 8(3): E443–49.

Thangapazham, R.L. et al. 2007. "Beneficial role of curcumin in skin diseases." *Advances in Experimental Medicine and Biology* 595:343–57.

Tsui, K.H. et al. 2008. "Curcumin blocks the activating of androgen and interlukin-6 on prostate specific antigen expression in human prostatic carcinoma cells." *Journal of Andrology* Jul 31 (Epub ahead of print).

Wang, X. et al. 2006. "Curcumin inhibits neurotensin-mediated interleukin-8 production and migration of HCT116 human colon cancer cells." *Clinical Cancer Research* 12(18): 5346–55.

World Health Organization. 1999. "WHO Monographs on Selected Medicinal Plants". Volume 1. Geneva: World Health Organization.

Yodkeeree S. et al. 2008. "Curcumin, demethoxycurcumin and bisdemethoxycurcumin differentially inhibit cancer cell invasion through the down-regulation of MMPs and uPA." *Journal of Nutritional Biochemistry* May 19 (Epub ahead of print).

About the Author

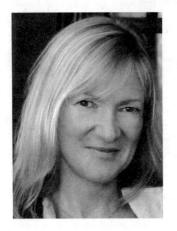

Barbara Wexler is a medical writer and chronic disease epidemiologist who brings more than 25 years of experience as a clinician, researcher, educator and administrator to the articles and texts she prepares for professional and consumer audiences. A graduate of Sarah Lawrence College and the Yale University College of Medicine, School of Epidemiology and Public Health, Wexler is interested in evidence-based complementary and integrative medicine.